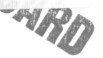

Gotta Minute?

The Ultimate Guide of One-Minute Workouts

for Anyone, Anywhere, Anytime!

by Bonnie Nygard, M.Ed.
and Bonnie Hopper, M.Ed

Robert D. Reed Publishers, San Francisco, CA

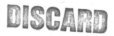

Robert D. Reed Publishers
750 La Playa Street, Suite 647
San Francisco, CA 94121
Phone: 650/994-6570
Fax: 650/994-6579
Email: 4bobreed@msn.com
Website: www.rdrpublishers.com

Editing and Typesetting by Betty Meyer
Illustrations by John McGee
Cover design by Julia A. Gaskill
  at Graphics Plus, Pacifica, California 94044

ISBN 1-885003-37-4
Library of Congress Card Number: 99-067464

Manufactured and printed in the United States.

Dedicated, with love, to our children Jeb, Katie, Corey, Shauna, Cole, and Hali.

Acknowledgments

Thanks to the dedicated researchers who conducted the *Project Active* study. This research focused on the effects of lifestyle activity versus structured aerobic exercise on sedentary adults and gave us the inspiration to write this book.

Love and appreciation to our families, friends, and students who provided support, creative ideas, and willing bodies to try out our lifestyle exercises with good humor and honest feedback.

This book would not have been possible without the dedication and hard work of John McGee, our talented illustrator, and Betty Meyer, who formatted and painstakingly assisted with editing the text. Thank you both!

An especially warm note of appreciation to Robert D. Reed, our publisher, who had confidence in this book and provided us with his valuable insights and expertise every step of the way.

Table of Contents

Introduction

Have you heard the saying "Inch by inch, it's a cinch. Yard by yard, it's too hard"? This quote can be directly applied to your own exercise habits and fitness level. We're going to show you how improving your health and physical fitness is a process whereby each small step (or minute of exercise) can take you closer to a better **quality of life**. Fortunately, research now supports the notion that exercise does not have to be time consuming or difficult in order to be effective. Improving your health and fitness can be a cinch!

The most common barriers to exercising are lack of time, lack of social support, inclement weather, disruptions in routine, lack of access to facilities, and a dislike of vigorous exercise. Following are exercise strategies that will help you overcome each of these barriers.

- **Lack of Time**: *Gotta Minute* will show you how to incorporate quick, easy, and effective exercises into your daily routine. It will take very little, if any, time out of your schedule. Most of the exercises are performed while doing daily tasks, such as talking on the phone, grocery shopping, doing laundry, etc.

- **Lack of Social Support:** Exercises outlined in *Gotta Minute* can be done inconspicuously. You can keep your program completely to yourself. Some of the exercises can be done with a partner or children in order to be inclusive. Social support is not an issue – this book alone provides support with light humor and very sound advice.

- **Inclement Weather:** All exercises in *Gotta Minute* can be done indoors. They do not depend on the weather.

- **Disruptions in Routine:** *Gotta Minute* provides exercise ideas that will be done during your regular routine. They will not disrupt your routine, just enhance it!

- **Lack of Access to Facilities:** Exercises described in *Gotta Minute* do not require special facilities. The emphasis is on performing exercises in your home, while you shop, in a car, at work, etc.

- **Dislike of Vigorous Exercise:** *Gotta Minute* is not a vigorous exercise program. It focuses on short, moderate-intensity exercises.

Gotta Minute offers a program that will allow you to reap the benefits of exercise without being confronted by any of the most common barriers. You will learn easy, fun, and quick ways to improve your health and well being.

If you're wondering how this can be true, here's your answer. Current research indicates that even short bouts of moderate exercise can have a very positive impact on your overall health AND improve physical fitness! In fact, studies have been conducted on the effects of infusing more movement and exercise into a person's daily routine. The results are very encouraging. Researchers found that including even short bouts of exercise into one's daily life can be as effective as a structured program for people who are not regularly active. Specifically, the research says that you can improve your level of physical activity, cardiorespiratory fitness, body composition, and reduce your blood pressure by simply adding more movement into what you already do during the day!

If your goal is to improve your cardiorespiratory fitness, body composition, and/or reduce your blood pressure, it is recommended you accumulate 30 minutes of exercise on most days of the week. As with any new exercise program, check with your physician to make sure the exercises are appropriate for you.

This book is divided into sections based on activities that most people do on a regular basis during their daily routine. Each section will share *"Fitness Facts"* that highlight interesting facts about exercise and fitness. In each section, you will receive basic exercise recommendations; instructions on how to perform your ONE-MINUTE workout exercises safely; and, when necessary, exercise modifications and choices for a variety of fitness levels. This book is written in no specific order. Begin with the section of your choice. In addition to improving your fitness and activity level, it is important to have fun and enjoy the process!

You may do some activities every day, or once a week, or less frequently. Do not try to adopt all of the activity ideas suggested in this book at once. Select one or two activities and become comfortable adding them to your daily routine. Then gradually add one activity at a time. In order for you to keep track of the exercises you are using, we have included an exercise log. Take a few moments to write down ONE-MINUTE workouts you are doing each day and/or week. This will act as a quick reminder and help keep you focused on your path to better health. The goal is for these ONE-MINUTE workouts to become an effortless part of your regular routine. Follow these simple suggestions and you will be amazed at the results. You will improve the quality of each day - **feel better**, **look better**, and **enjoy life**! Let's get started!

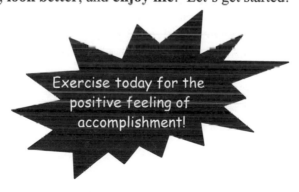

Exercise today for the positive feeling of accomplishment!

Fitness Fact: In 1996, the Surgeon General's Report on Physical Activity and Health reported that significant improvements in health and life expectancy can be obtained through moderate increases in physical activity. This report also states that physical activity need not be strenuous to achieve health benefits.

Getting Started!

In order for this, or any exercise program to work for you, you must do the following:

- **Do it for yourself** and believe that you are worth it! No matter what else is going on in your life, you deserve to take better care of your health and well being.

- **Monitor your success** by how you feel and how much more energy you have, not by the number on the scale! Remember that this program is designed to accommodate your daily schedule ONE-MINUTE at a time. Enjoy the new focus on being active throughout the day and the rest will follow.

- **Don't rush it** People who try to do too much, too soon, tend to burn out on an exercise program. Take it one step, and ONE-MINUTE, at a time. This book will introduce you to a whole new way of approaching daily activities. Take it slowly and have fun!

- **Set realistic and action-oriented goals** Goal setting is a very powerful motivator and will help you identify obstacles before they can get in your way. Rome wasn't built in a day. The same is true for your exercise goals. Make sure your expectations are realistic. This book will help you achieve your goals one step at a time. In order to achieve your goals, you must be willing to work for them. What action are you willing to take to achieve your goals? The exercises in this book can be the 'action!'

An example of a goal is:

My Exercise Goal is *to feel better, have more energy, and less stress.*

My action plan for achieving this goal is *to give myself ONE-MINUTE workouts throughout the day in order to increase my exercise level to 20 minutes per day.*

I will benefit from accomplishing this goal by *having more confidence, being able to do more during the day without feeling tired, and being in a better and more relaxed mood.*

Review your goal from time to time and always give it positive energy!

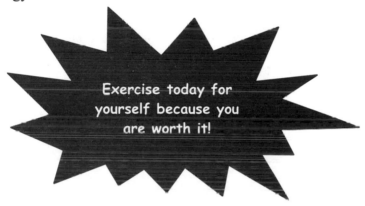

Exercise today for
yourself because you
are worth it!

We have included a goal setting chart for you to complete. Please take a moment and fill this out.

ONE-MINUTE Workout Goal!
"If it's going to be, it's up to me!"

NAME: _____ **DATE:** _____

My Exercise Goal is: *(i.e., have more energy throughout the day)* _____

_____

My Action Plan for achieving this goal is: *(i.e., use one-minute activities four days per week)* _____

_____

I will benefit from accomplishing my goal by: *(i.e., having more energy)* ____

_____

The following people and/or groups will help me accomplish my goal: *(i.e., family, co-workers, friends, etc.)* _____

_____

I will overcome the following obstacles in order to achieve my goal: *(i.e, the mindset that I can't improve my fitness)* _____

_____

I will accomplish my goal by this date: _____

I will give my exercise goals positive energy every day! I will overcome obstacles and challenges that may keep me from attaining my goals!

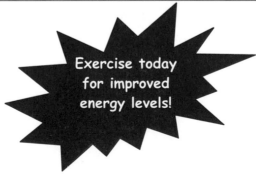

Exercise today
for improved
energy levels!

One-Minute Workout
Log and Daily Diary

We have included a ONE-MINUTE Workout Log in this book for your use. This will help you keep track of the exercises you are already doing, allowing you to take pride in your accomplishments, and stay motivated "minute" to "minute." It also provides you with an opportunity to reflect on how you feel and will show you how easy it is to accumulate workout minutes using this program. Before you know it, you'll be exercising 15-30 minutes per day and feeling great!

If you enjoy keeping a daily diary, we have also included a ONE–MINUTE Workout Diary. We recommend you use the ONE-MINUTE Workout Log for the first several weeks. Once you accumulate a minimum of 15 exercise minutes per day, move on to the daily diary. Keep track of all of the exercises you are doing each day for an entire week and be amazed at how fast your exercise minutes add up! **Feel free to copy these daily diary pages** and continue to keep your exercise diary for as long as you wish. It's a great way to reflect on your exercise accomplishments.

Fitness Fact: Health-related physical fitness includes five components: cardiorespiratory (aerobic) fitness, muscular endurance, muscular strength, body composition, and flexibility. We believe there is a sixth component to health-related fitness, and that is stress management. What do you think?

One-Minute Workout Log!
"Where you come from
isn't as important as where you are going."

ONE-MINUTE Workouts Currently in use: *Example:* *Toothbrush heel raises*	How Often per Week/Day: *2 per day*	Average Min. per Day: *2 Min.*	Workout Comments: *Easy to do. My calf muscles* *feel stronger.*

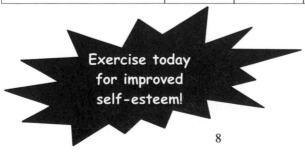

Exercise today
for improved
self-esteem!

One-Minute Workout Log!
"Seven days without exercise makes one WEAK."

ONE-MINUTE Workouts Currently in use:	How Often per Week/Day:	Average Min. per Day:	Workout Comments:

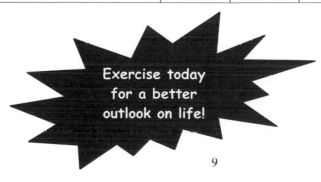

Exercise today
for a better
outlook on life!

One-Minute Workout Log!
"If you're headed in the right direction, each step, no matter how small, is getting you closer to your goal!"

ONE-MINUTE Workouts Currently in use:	How Often per Week/Day:	Average Min. per Day:	Workout Comments:

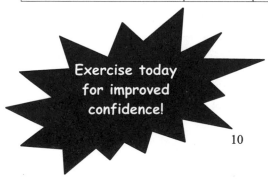

Exercise today for improved confidence!

The ONE-MINUTE Workout Diary!

SUNDAY

ONE-MINUTE Workouts: *Example: Laundry Basket Presses*	Minutes: *3 Min.*
TOTAL Workout Minutes:	
Comments:	

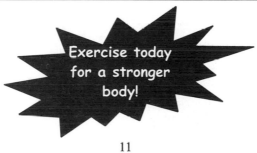

Exercise today for a stronger body!

The ONE-MINUTE Workout Diary!

MONDAY

ONE-MINUTE Workouts: *Example: Lunch Hour Walk*	Minutes: *5 Min.*
TOTAL Workout Minutes:	

Comments:

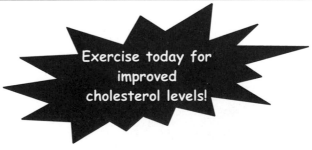

Exercise today for
improved
cholesterol levels!

The ONE-MINUTE Workout Diary!

TUESDAY

ONE-MINUTE Workouts: *Example: Aerobic Shopping*	Minutes: *10 Min.*
TOTAL Workout Minutes:	
Comments:	

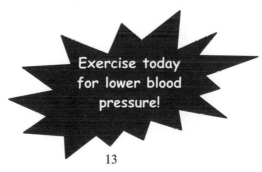

Exercise today
for lower blood
pressure!

The ONE-MINUTE Workout Diary!

WEDNESDAY

ONE-MINUTE Workouts: *Example: Upper Body TV Workout*	Minutes: *20 Min.*
TOTAL Workout Minutes:	
Comments:	

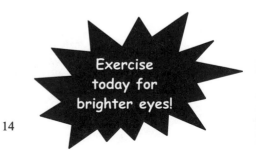

Exercise today for brighter eyes!

14

The ONE-MINUTE Workout Diary!

THURSDAY

ONE-MINUTE Workouts: *Example: Computer Workouts*	Minutes: *10 Min.*
TOTAL Workout Minutes:	
Comments:	

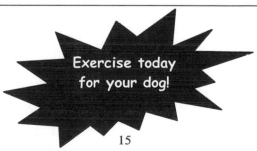

Exercise today
for your dog!

The ONE-MINUTE Workout Diary!

FRIDAY

ONE-MINUTE Workouts: *Example: Table Setting Curls*	Minutes: *3 Min.*
TOTAL Workout Minutes:	
Comments:	

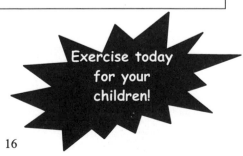

Exercise today
for your
children!

The ONE-MINUTE Workout Diary!

SATURDAY

ONE-MINUTE Workouts: *Example: Healthy Heart TV Workout*	Minutes: *20 Min.*
TOTAL Workout Minutes:	
Comments:	

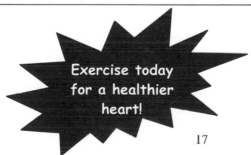

Exercise today
for a healthier
heart!

Muscle Charts

These muscle charts are quick-and-easy muscle anatomy references. We recommend you select exercises from this book that work a variety of muscles. You will notice, throughout this book, we provide you with the scientific names of muscles. These charts will provide you with the location of each of those muscles.

Front

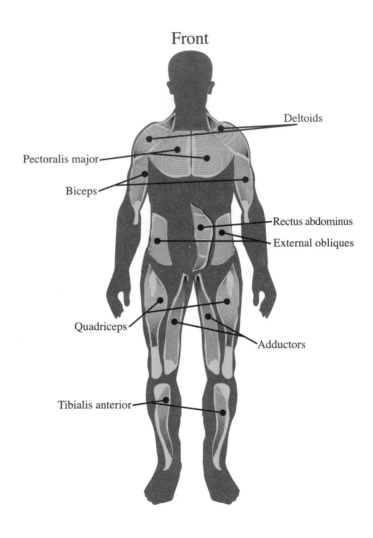

Back

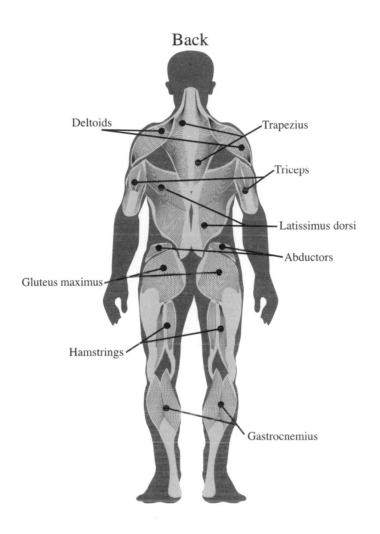

Deltoids

Trapezius

Triceps

Latissimus dorsi

Abductors

Gluteus maximus

Hamstrings

Gastrocnemius

ONE-MINUTE
Everyday Workouts!

Fitness Fact: The most important "Power Food" is not even food at all. It's water! Dehydration reduces energy. Your daily intake of water should be approximately half your body weight in ounces. For example, if you weigh 160 lb., you should drink 80 ounces of water every day. There are eight ounces in a cup, so that would be approximately 10 cups of water per day. Okay…the extra energy you'll experience is well worth the little extra bathroom time!

This section introduces a variety of ways in which you can incorporate exercise into your everyday routine. If you have a roommate or live with your family, invite them to participate in your one-minute workouts. This can provide you with very valuable social support in your own home. Better yet, you can support one another while having some fun with your everyday exercises! And, you're bound to create even more one-minute workouts. Cheer each other on and be committed to creating a better quality of life in your household.

Exercise today for less stress!

Rise & Shine Stretches

So you've hit the snooze button seven times already! Don't leap out of bed into a potentially stressful day. First, take ONE more minute and perform the following relaxing and effective *Rise & Shine Stretches*:

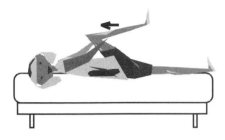

Lying on your back, bend your right knee and gently lift it toward your chest and hold for a slow count of ten. Hold your leg in place with hands placed on your thigh (under your knee), not over your knee (this places stress on your knee). Breathe deeply throughout the stretch. Repeat the same stretch with your left leg. This is oh so good for your lower back!

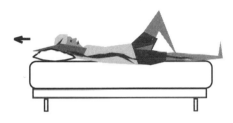

Extend your right leg straight down onto the bed and place the left foot on the bed with a bent knee. Extend your right arm over your head and stretch your arm upward while stretching your right leg down (in opposite directions). This is a fabulous full-body stretch. Reverse the stretch you just completed. Bend your right knee and place that foot on the bed. Stretch your left leg down and your left arm up. Ahhh.... Now, you're ready for the day!

Bed Laps
Instead of reaching across the bed to make it, walk around the bed to finish the job. You'll burn a few extra calories and save your back from the potential strain of reaching to the other side.

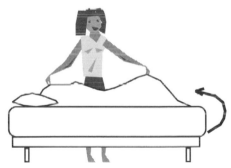

Exercise today for a better night's sleep!

21

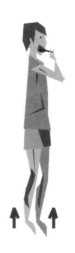

Tooth Brushing Heel Raises

Turn polishing your pearly whites into a heel raising experience! Stand with feet a little more than hip distance apart and slowly raise and lower your heels off the floor. This is a fantastic exercise for sculpting your calf muscles (gastrocnemius).

Flossing Toe Taps

Now that you've worked those calves while brushing, let's balance the workout as you floss. While flossing your upper teeth, do toe taps with your right foot; do toe taps with the left foot while flossing your lower teeth. This works the front side of your shins (tibialis anterior) which are often neglected.

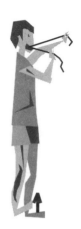

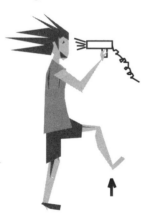

Balance & Blow-Dry

Alternate balancing on one foot and then the other while blow-drying or combing your hair. Many lower body muscles will be working to help improve your balance!

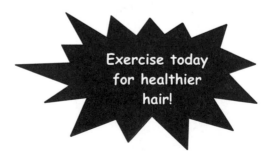

Exercise today
for healthier
hair!

22

A Hip Way to Read the Paper

In-between newspaper articles or pages, stand, raise one foot off the floor and perform large circles with your lifted leg by bringing it to the front, side, and back of your body. This is excellent for improving range of motion in your hips, and works a variety of leg and trunk muscles. If you need a little help with balance, hold the back of a chair or countertop while performing this exercise.

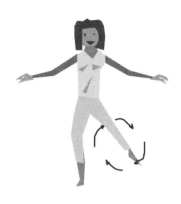

Chapter Changes

Don't worry, we won't suggest giving up your time to relax with a good book. Relax and savor each chapter. When you complete a chapter, set the book down and rotate your hands in small circles (using your wrists), first to the right and then to the left, the number that corresponds with the next chapter. For example, if you just completed

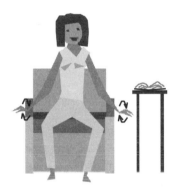

Chapter Five and are about to begin Chapter Six, perform six hand circles in each direction and then pick up your book and resume reading. This exercise improves range of motion in your wrists and stimulates sleepy hands!

Phone Fitness Talking on the phone doesn't have to be "down" time. Pick UP the phone, catch UP with a friend, and add the *TRI-Umph* exercises for an UP beat mini workout! The following three exercises target muscles that are generally very weak. This can result in low back pain and posture malalignments. Once you see how easy these exercises are, they will become a regular part of your phone conversations! We're not recommending a specific number of repetitions for these exercises because you'll be too busy talking to count. Instead, do as many repetitions as are comfortable. If you're a *phone person* (you know if you are!), repeat the exercises only to the point of muscular fatigue, never to the point of pain. (This is the key to improving one's endurance and strength in any muscle group.)

Begin by doing only *Gluteal Contractions* throughout your conversation. When next on the phone, do *Ab Busters*, and then move on to *Shoulder Squeezes* on the next call. Once you can easily combine each of these *TRI-Umph* exercises with your phone conversations, mix them up and alternate doing all three during the same conversation. You will be TRI-umphant!

"TRI-Umph!"

Gluteal Contractions – Alternate squeezing, holding a few seconds, then relaxing your buttocks (gluteus maximus). Repeat as many times as you like and, if time permits, move on to the *Ab Busters*. Keep breathing, and talking, throughout the exercises.

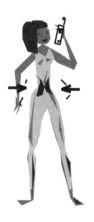

Ab Busters – Alternate contracting, holding, then relaxing your stomach, or abdominal muscles. To contract these muscles, attempt to bring your navel (belly button) toward your spine. Continue to breathe throughout the exercise and keep the conversation going. It does take some extra concentration, but we know you're up to the challenge!

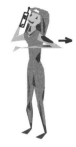

Shoulder Blade Squeezes – Bring your shoulder blades together in back and then relax them. Again, breathe throughout the exercise while opening up your chest and shoulders. This works your upper back muscles (trapezius and rhomboids) and feels great! Plus, your posture is benefited.

Avoid the Bills

Instead of walking directly to your mailbox to retrieve the mail, avoid those bills for an extra minute by extending your walk to your neighbor's mailbox. Then, return to your own mailbox, retrieve your mail, and face the music! Once this becomes a daily habit, extend your mailbox trek, one neighbor at a time, until you're walking around the entire block. It sure beats paying bills!

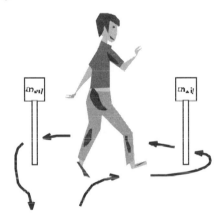

ONE-MINUTE
Grocery Shopping Workouts!

Fitness Fact: Feeling stressed out? Exercise can help control the negative effects of stress. Hormones, called endorphins, are released during exercise that provide a relaxation response and improve your mood. Exercise helps you feel better about yourself and reduces anxiety. Last, but not least, people who exercise regularly tend to eat healthier foods. Good nutrition assists your body to control the negative effects of stress. Keep this in mind as you shop.

Have you ever gone to the grocery store on an empty stomach and ended up with a cart overflowing with all your favorite, not-so-healthy foods? As you begin adding up your one-minute workouts, this will be less likely to occur because exercising can actually depress your appetite! In addition, taking along some bottled water (or buying one) and drinking as you shop will keep you hydrated and will suppress your appetite.

This section will introduce you to some fun ways to add short exercises before, during, and after grocery shopping. And, by the way, it's okay to treat yourself to some decadent food choices from time to time – in MODERATION! Going out for a thin slice of cheesecake can be a reward for reaching your goal of exercising 20 minutes per day and sticking with it for a month!

If your goal is to lose a few pounds, begin by drinking plenty of water (at least 10 glasses per day) and do NOT go on a fad diet. Healthy, permanent weight loss is a gradual process – you should not attempt to lose more than one to two pounds per week. A healthy diet includes 55-60% of your daily calories in the form of carbohydrates (grains, pasta, rice, vegetables, fruits, etc.), 10-12% in the form of protein (lean meats, beans, skinless poultry, etc.), and less than 30% in the form of fat. Never skip meals. Avoid laxatives and/or diuretics. Exercise your way to safe and effective weight loss.

Parking Space Shuffle

Instead of parking in the closest space, park in the 2nd closest parking space and walk that little extra to the store entrance. As you become accustomed to the extra walking distance, park in the 3rd, 4th, and 5th closest parking space. Eventually, you'll be walking the length of the parking lot on every trip. If you have children, involve them in the *"Parking Space Shuffle"* by allowing them to determine which space you'll park in that day.

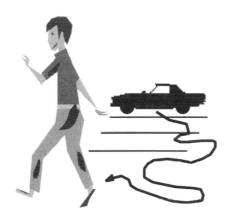

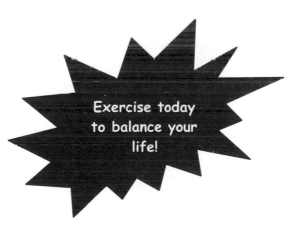

Exercise today to balance your life!

Get Your Cart, Get Set, SHOP!
Before getting into some serious grocery shopping, take a minute and walk one lap around the perimeter of the store. Watch out for other shoppers as you round those corners!

Shelf Stretches and Lunges

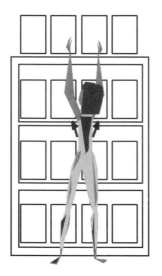

Instead of reaching for an item on an upper shelf with one hand, extend both arms and get a shoulder and upper back stretch out of the process.

For items (non-glass, please) that are waist high, collect them from behind your back. That's right, walk up to the shelf, turn your back to the item and reach your arm back and nab it. Alternate your right and left arm.

This provides a much-needed stretch for your chest (pectorals) and the front of your shoulders (anterior deltoids). Worried about looking goofy? Humor is a very powerful stress reliever. Don't be afraid to have some fun and get a chuckle out of your new activities. At the same time, you'll probably help some other shoppers with their stress level!

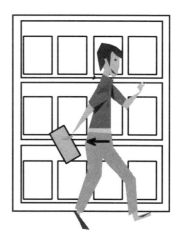

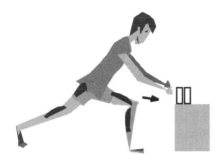

For those items on the lower shelves, don't bend at the waist (this places stress on your back). Take a big step forward with one foot and slowly lower your body into a lunge. (Keep your front knee directly above your front ankle for safe alignment). Take your time by s-l-o-w-l-y lunging down and then slowly standing up. Balance the workout by alternating your lead leg for each lunge, or better yet, perform two lunges (one with your right leg in front and one with your left leg in front) for every item retrieved from a lower shelf. It's a great way to work your lower body (gluteals, hamstrings, and quadriceps)!

The Dreaded Line
Don't fret if you find yourself standing in a checkout line where you need binoculars to see the clerk. Try one, or all, of the following inconspicuous exercises, and no one will ever suspect you are giving yourself a mini-workout: (Add a little "Umph!" and you will be triumphant!)

"TRI-Umph!"

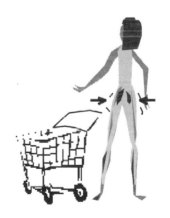

Gluteal Contractions – Contract your buttocks (gluteus maximus) and hold for a slow count of four and then release for a slow count of four. Try to do eight repetitions (each repetition includes a four-count contraction and a four-count release or relax phase) before you get to the front of the line. Keep breathing throughout the exercise and think about how nice it will be to have buns that feel like hard metal! Yes, you can have a conversation with someone while doing this. (Okay, you may need a little practice!)

29

Ab Busters - Contract your stomach, or abdominal muscles, and hold for a slow count of four and then release for a slow count of four. Try to do eight repetitions before you get to the front of the line. Keep breathing throughout the exercise. Feel free to converse with a friend or family member during this exercise.

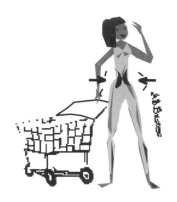

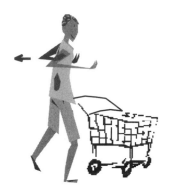

Shoulder Blade Squeezes – Press your shoulder blades together in back and hold for a slow count of four and then release for a slow count of four. Try to do eight repetitions before you get to the front of the line. Keep breathing throughout the exercise. Again, converse with others and enjoy the experience. This is a great exercise for improving a rounded shoulder posture.

Home Again, Home Again
Remove your groceries from your car, two bags at a time and perform biceps curls with a bag in each hand as you transfer them into your house. Now that you have curled all the groceries into the house, it's time to put them away.

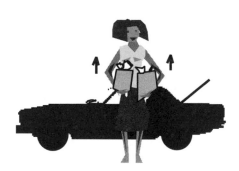

Use the same *Shelf Stretches and Lunges* that you performed at the grocery store. This time, perform them to put your groceries away at home. Wow, that feels good!

ONE-MINUTE
Household Workouts!

Fitness Fact: Exercise builds muscle mass, which increases metabolic rate, even during inactivity. In other words, exercise helps you burn more calories even while you rest!

Have you ever thought of housecleaning as a real workout? If your answer is "yes," you're right! A person weighing 160 lb. burns approximately 200 calories in one hour of light housecleaning. Just think of the extra calories you can burn by adding a little "extra" to your chores. This section is devoted to helping you do just that. Don't be surprised if you find your fingers dialing up a friend to see if you can assist them with their household workout. Look out!

Exercise today because it's fun!

Aerobic House Cleaning!

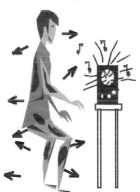

Before getting into the real chores at hand, turn on and crank up your favorite upbeat music and boogie off a few extra calories while you clean. If you're ready for an extra challenge, try vacuuming, sweeping, and dusting to the beat. Strive to go non-stop for five minutes or more, keeping those legs moving. YAAHOOO!

VaVOOM-Vacuum!

You probably always use the same arm to push your vacuum cleaner. Switch your pushing arm on every 8th push and balance

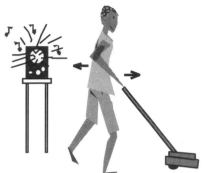

the workout. This will give the front of your shoulder (anterior deltoids) and back of your shoulder (posterior deltoids) an equal workout. Give that machine a real push (triceps) and pull (biceps) to tone your arm muscles. Voom! Voom! VaVOOM!

Mopping with Meaning

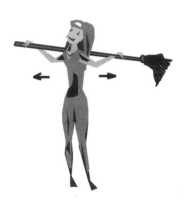

While mopping, alternate hand positions on the handle and balance the workout. Believe it or not, a mop handle can also be an excellent piece of exercise equipment. Place the mop across your shoulders (behind your head), holding it in place with arms extended out to the sides. Perform slow and gentle twists, moving your shoulders to the right and then left. This is great for your spine and obliques. Life does tend to throw twists at you; exercising will help you be ready for them!

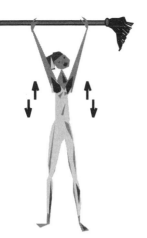

You can also take that mop and perform some shoulder presses. Holding the mop in front of your upper body with your hands about shoulder-width apart, slowly press the mop above your head and then lower it. Exhale as you lift and inhale as you lower the mop. This works your shoulder muscles (deltoids).

You can also check out your level of hip flexibility with a mop handle. Hold the handle in front of your lower body, with hands shoulder-width apart, and slightly bend your knees. Attempt to step both legs over the handle with one leg at a time, without releasing the mop handle! If you are able to step over the handle with both legs, step one leg at a time back through to the start position. This might be a challenge and a half! You're not a bad person if you can't do it, just work on improving your flexibility.

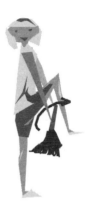

Broom Alert!

If you use a broom, don't sweep these exercises under the rug. Every mop exercise can be performed with a broom!

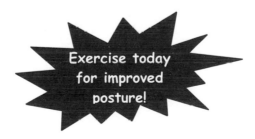

Exercise today for improved posture!

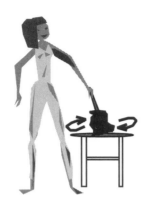

Dusting Twirls

Turn your dusting into an equal opportunity workout by changing dusting hands, twirling the dust rag eight times in each direction before changing hands. Before you know it, you'll see sculpted arm muscles in your tabletop shine!

Laundry Basket Squats

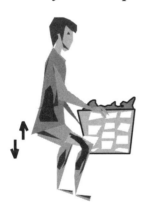

We already know that doing laundry can be a real chore. By making a few adjustments, you can turn this chore into a choice workout! When bending to pick up your laundry basket, bend at the hips and squat down using your legs. Check to see that your knees stay in safe alignment, and are directly above your ankles. Lean your upper body only a little forward. Pick up the basket, bring it close to your body, and then stand. This is great for your buttocks (gluteals) and thigh muscles (quadriceps and hamstrings) AND protects your back. If you're up to the challenge, repeat this several times (eight?) with each lift.

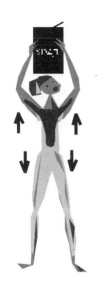

Laundry Detergent Presses

When doing laundry, you may have to pick up a container (bottle or box) of laundry detergent. You can turn this simple task into a military press and get a great chest (pectorals), shoulder (deltoids), and arm (triceps) workout! Hold the detergent or bleach container with both of your hands, in front of your body. Now, raise the container slowly by pushing it up (with both arms) over your head, then lowering it slowly. Repeat this four to eight times for each load of laundry. You'll get a double-weight workout if you use both detergent and bleach. Again, breathe (exhale as you lift the detergent, inhale as you lower) throughout each exercise and take the upward press and lowering phase slowly. If you are only able to do one or two presses, that's okay. Each step will get you closer to your goal!

Now that you've got the detergent in the machine, let's work on getting those dirty clothes in. Each time you put a handful of clothes in the machine, perform alternating leg extensions to the back of your body. Simply raise one leg to the back approximately 10-12 inches and then return the leg to start position. Try to keep the leg you are lifting straight (not bent), keep your back straight (not arched), and abdominal muscles tight. By doing so, you protect your lower back. Now, do this with the other leg. Repeat one to four times (or more) with each leg.

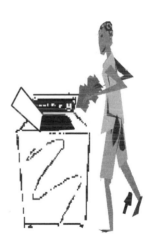

This works your gluteus maximus (buttocks)…your "rear view."

Upper Body Towel Stretches (Pain = NO Gain!)

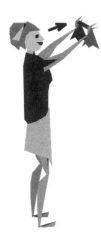

To conclude your laundry workout, take a few seconds out of your folding time and give yourself some much-needed stretches! It is very important to hold your stretches only to the point of comfortable tension, never to the point of pain. When your brain receives a pain message from a muscle, it sends a message back telling the muscle to contract in order to protect itself. Effective stretching occurs when the muscles are relaxed, not contracted. Breathe slowly and relax into each stretch.

Take a bath or kitchen towel and hold an opposite end in each hand so your arms are shoulder-width apart.

(1) While holding the towel, extend your arms over and slightly in front of your head – stretching your shoulders and back muscles (lats or latissimus dorsi muscle). Hold this stretch for a slow count of ten. Remember to breathe.

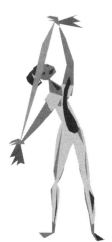

(2) Lower your right hand to the side. This will cause your left hand to extend over your head – stretching the left side of your body (obliques). Hold for a count of ten and enjoy. Repeat to the other side. You're not holding your breath, are you?

(3) Bring both arms straight out in front of your chest, slightly round your back, and hold for a count of ten – stretching your upper-back muscles (trapezius and rhomboids).

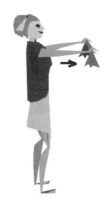

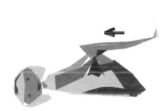

(4) Drop one end of your towel in order to bring it behind your back. Holding each end with hands behind your back, raise the towel slightly upward and hold for a count of ten – stretching your chest (pectorals) and shoulders (anterior or front deltoids).

Lower Body Towel Stretches

(1) Lying on your back, place the towel under your thighs, and hold opposite ends of the towel in each hand. Slowly bend your knees and lift them toward your chest. Assist this process with your towel. Keep your head and shoulders on the floor or you will be placing strain on your neck. Hold this position for a slow count of ten – stretching your low back muscles (erector spinae).

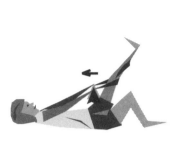

(2) From the same position, place the towel under your right thigh and place your other foot on the floor (knee bent). Lift the towel-wrapped leg up and toward your body, keeping the leg straight – stretching the back of that leg (hamstrings). Hold for a slow count of ten and repeat with your left leg. Did you know that tight hamstrings are directly related to lower back pain? It's true. By stretching your hamstrings, you are caring for your lower back as well!

Iron Away Those Saddlebags

For you non-horse lovers who wish to remove the saddlebags attached to your outer thighs, here's a chore you can't ignore! While ironing your clothes, slowly raise and lower one leg at a time to the side of your body. Try to keep your body upright as you perform these side leg-raises and breathe through each exercise. You can do this without missing a wrinkle – keep ironing. "Hay", this will tone your outer thighs (abductors)!

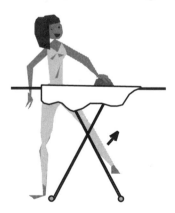

ONE-MINUTE
Cooking Workouts!

Fitness Fact: Exercises performed slowly are more beneficial than those done quickly. When you perform an exercise slowly, momentum no longer assists the process and your muscle is required to work harder and longer.

For a healthy diet, the U.S. Departments of Agriculture and Health and Human Services recommend eating a variety of foods; balancing the food you eat with physical activity; choosing a diet low in fat, sugars, and salt; and choosing a diet with plenty of grain products, vegetables, and fruits. Listed below are a few tips to help you achieve a healthy, more varied diet.

- Before shopping, plan your meals for the week and include the different food groups (grains, fruits, vegetables, protein, and dairy).
- Buy a healthy cooking cookbook and try new meal combinations.
- Gather a list of different fruits, vegetables, and grains and create a meal around one or more of them each week.
- Try a new restaurant that serves healthy food you've never tried.

Now that you have some ideas on how to plan an exciting meal, here are some creative ways to include exercise in the culinary process!

Cupboard Stretches and Lunges
Just like at the grocery store, when reaching for an item and/or dish from an upper shelf, extend both arms and get a shoulder and upper back stretch out of the process.

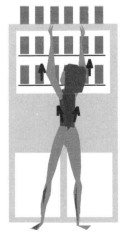

39

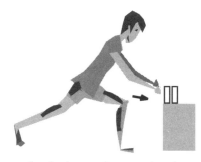

You can transform collecting items and/or cooking utensils from your lower cupboards into a lower body workout. To retrieve those items, don't bend forward at the waist (this places stress on your back). Use your legs. Take a big step forward with one foot and slowly lower your body into a lunge. Again, maintain safe alignment by keeping the front knee directly above the ankle. Take your time by s-l-o-w-l-y lunging down and then slowly standing up. Yep, you're working those gluteals, hamstrings, and quadriceps.

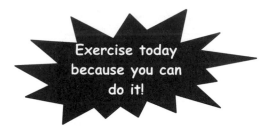

Exercise today because you can do it!

Any CAN Can!

Does your cooking involve opening a can or two? That's okay, because any CAN can give you a mini-biceps workout! Before opening, hold the can with palm facing up. Now, lift the can toward your shoulder by bending your elbow. Keep your elbow close to your side as you curl the can up, repeat eight times, and then transfer the can to your other hand and do eight curls on that side. Exhale as you lift the can and inhale as you lower. Remember, do this slowly in both directions for the most benefit!

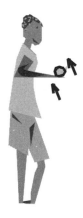

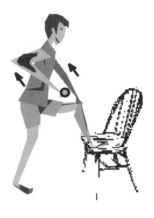

Here's a great "can" exercise for your back (lats and trapezius). Hold the can in one hand and place the opposite foot on a kitchen chair, resting your free hand on your lifted thigh or on the chair for balance. Now, lift the bent elbow of the arm that's holding the can up and back (like starting a lawnmower in slow motion). Exhale as you lift the elbow back and up, and inhale as you lower it slowly to start position.

These exercises will also work with a bag of rice, flour, pasta, dog food, etc. Create your own resistance exercises while you heat it up in the kitchen. Remember this only takes seconds out of your cooking time.

You're Getting HOTTER!

While standing by the stove, heat up your lower body by alternating heel and toe raises. Stand with your feet a little more than hip-width apart (for good stability and balance) and slowly rock back on your heels and raise your toes off the floor – this works the front side of your lower legs (tibialis anterior). Now, shift your weight forward to your toes and raise your heels off the floor – this works your calf muscles (gastrocnemius). You can alternate raising toes and heels or do eight repetitions of each before changing from one to the other. For best results, try to perform these exercises in a slow and 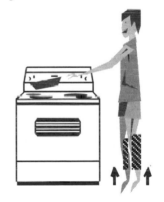 controlled manner. Again, breathe, enjoy, and only exercise to the point of fatigue, never to the point of pain. In addition to shaping your lower legs, this exercise is great for improving balance. For a greater challenge, lift one foot off the floor and perform toe and heel raises while balancing on one foot. Wow!

Table Setting Curls

While setting your table for a meal, perform leg curls as you walk.

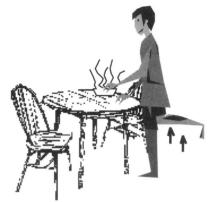

Since you're already moving, you might as well make the most of it and get a great hamstring workout while you set. This also works while clearing the dirty dishes. This exercise may feel awkward at first, but give it a chance and you'll love the overall effect. The hamstring muscles tend to be neglected throughout the day so they will appreciate your effort!

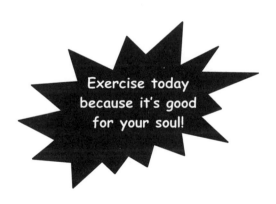

Exercise today because it's good for your soul!

ONE-MINUTE
Computer Workouts!

Before getting into the specific computer exercises, here are some tips for healthy posture while sitting in a chair. When asked to do a posture check, think of the following "Sitting Rules":

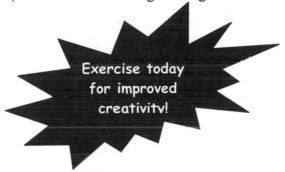

Sitting Rules

- Sit with your head in line with your spine. Your chin should not protrude forward.
- Aim to have your knees slightly higher than your hips.
- Do not slump back in your chair, instead sit slightly forward.
- When reaching for something while sitting, bend forward from the hips to retrieve the item.
- Make sure your chair offers lower back support. If it doesn't, use a rolled towel and adjust it throughout each sitting in order to assure it is providing support to your lower back.
- After sitting for long periods of time (30 minutes or so), stand and stretch.

We know working on a computer can be somewhat complicated with all the new programs and technology available to us. To counter this, we've kept the computer exercises very easy and basic. Great care has been taken to provide you with exercises that are most needed when working on a computer for extended periods of time. It would be easy for us to tell you to perform specific exercises every ten minutes or so. This would also make it easy for you not to do them! So, we've devised common computer cues that will remind you when to do each exercise. Every time you perform each of the following "COMPUTER CUES," perform the associated "EXERCISE": (Before you know it, you'll have these memorized!)

COMPUTER CUE:

EXERCISE:

START UP (Turn it on & wait)

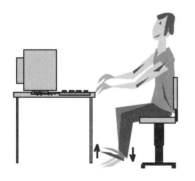

Rev up! While seated, alternate walking in place on your toes and heels (i.e. toes-toes, heel-heel, etc.). When you speed up this exercise, we believe it speeds up the software loading process! Continue until your computer is fired up. Adjust your chair for healthy posture and get to work!

SAVE or SEND (for e-mailers)

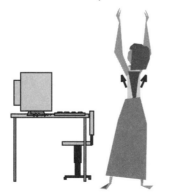

Stand, Squeeze, Stretch, and Sit! Stand up, squeeze your shoulder blades together. Stretch your arms up toward the ceiling while taking a deep breath. Sit down, adjust your chair for healthy posture, and get back to work!

44

OPEN (a file or program)

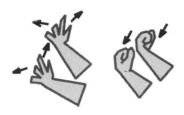

Open and close fingers. Spread your fingers open as wide as possible and then close them into a fist. Repeat four to eight times, check your sitting posture and get back to work. This is a great hand and forearm exercise. (For a little extra resistance, try this exercise with a rubber band wrapped around your fingers!)

NEW (creating anything new)

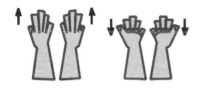

Knuckle bend. Extend your fingers straight up, with fingers close together. Now, bend them at the middle knuckles so they fold toward your palm. Repeat four to eight times, check your sitting posture and get back to work. Another great exercise for your busy hands and forearms.

PRINT

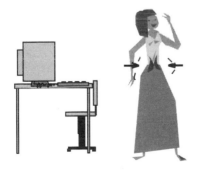

Posture check! This includes three simple exercises:

(1) Stand up and contract your abdominal muscles (pressing your navel toward your spine) and then relax your abdominal muscles;

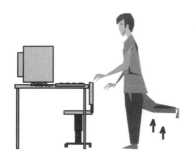

(2) Perform one to four alternating leg curls (lift your right foot up toward your buttocks and then your left foot) for stronger hamstrings; and

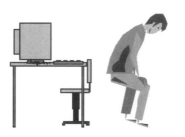

(3) Standing with slightly bent legs (using your hips to bend), place your hands on your thighs, bring your chin toward your chest, and round your back for an excellent low back stretch.
Sit down, check your posture and get back to work! Each of the three exercises listed above promotes healthy posture.

CLOSE (a document or program)

Close your eyes, inhale and exhale deeply, relax your hands, arms and shoulders. You sure needed that!

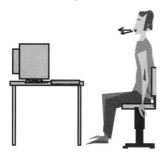

ONE-MINUTE
Out & About Workouts!

Fitness Fact: Did your mother ever tell you to "Stand up straight!"? Don't worry, the rounded shoulder posture is very common in both adolescents and adults, and can be caused by the way we live. Since much of what we do in our daily lives is done to the front of our bodies (driving, typing, carrying, lifting, etc.), our chest muscles (pectorals) are constantly being contracted throughout the day. This causes them to be short and tight. Conversely, our upper back muscles (trapezius) are being stretched throughout the day. This causes them to be over-stretched and weak. As a result, our short, tight chest muscles pull our shoulders forward while our over-stretched back muscles allow it to happen. This causes the rounded shoulder posture. Fortunately, there is hope! By stretching your chest and exercising, or contracting, your upper back muscles, you can improve your posture. You may have already noticed this book contains exercises that are designed to do just that.

Traveling can be an exciting adventure. Unfortunately, it can also be a sedentary experience. Long flights, car trips, or train rides can place us in a seated position with very limited space. This section includes exercises that can be performed while traveling. In addition, we'd like to share the following tips for adding exercise to your travels with little hassle:

- Before leaving home, find out if your hotel has an exercise facility or pool. If so, pack some loose, non-restrictive exercise clothes and/or a swimsuit.

- Never leave home without walking shoes!

- When you arrive at your destination, find out the location of nearby safe parks or recreational facilities where you can walk away any "down" time.

- Instead of ordering room service, ask for directions to a nearby eatery and walk to dinner.

Stairs Anyone?

When using the elevator, get off on the floor BELOW the one you wish to visit and walk up one flight. After you become comfortable doing this, get off two floors below your destination and walk two flights, etc. If you're confronted with stairs on a regular basis, mix it up by performing leg curls as you climb. This can turn stair climbing into a real kick!

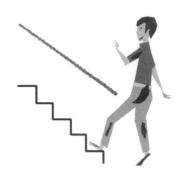

TRI-Umph!

Use the three *TRI-Umph* exercises whenever you find yourself in a line, i.e., at the bank, department store, public restroom (oh NO!), etc. Don't just stand there, contract something!

Car Calisthenics?

Okay, we won't have you do calisthenics in the car! But, before you drive on, be reminded of the following "Sitting Rules" for healthy posture:

- Sit with your head in line with your spine. Your chin should not protrude forward.

- Aim to have your knees slightly higher than your hips.

- Do not slump back in your seat, instead sit slightly forward.

- Make sure your car seat offers lower back support. If it doesn't, use a rolled towel and adjust it, when necessary, in order to assure it is providing support to your lower back.

Red Light-Green Light!
Any or all of the following exercises can be done while stopped at a red light:

- Reach both arms up and place your hands on the ceiling of your car. Breathe deeply and enjoy this shoulder stretch. Keep your foot on the brake, please!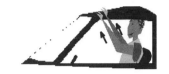

- Open fingers wide apart and then close them into a fist. Now, extend fingers straight up and then fold them, at the knuckles, toward your palm. Alternate these two exercises and try performing them quickly. This is a fun way to strengthen your hands and forearms!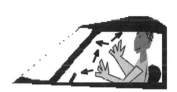

- Start with your shoulders back and lined up under your ears. Raise both shoulders up toward your ears and then relax. Perform each repetition slowly and continue to breathe throughout each exercise. This exercise is called shoulder shrugs and is a wonderful exercise for your neck and upper shoulders (upper trapezius/deltoids).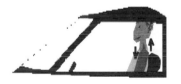

- Roll your shoulders backward and then toward the front. This is fabulous for relieving shoulder tension. Ahhh, that feels good.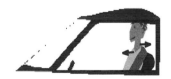

- You knew this one was coming! Contract your abdominal muscles (pressing your navel toward your spine) and hold for a slow count of four. Breathe throughout the exercise. Relax the abdominal muscles and repeat for as long as the light remains red.

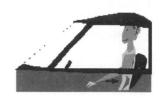

- Take advantage of one or two red lights and just relax. Rest your eyes (for only a moment at a time!), clear your mind of worries, and focus on feeling good about yourself. Don't worry, the car behind you will let you know when it's time to "Go!"

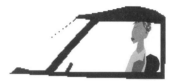

- If your commute provides you with numerous red lights, throw in some gluteal contractions and shoulder blade squeezes for more variety.

During green lights, drive safely!

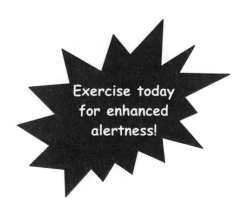

Exercise today for enhanced alertness!

Traffic Jam Blues

Find yourself in a traffic jam? Don't be blue. Use this opportunity to relax, breathe deeply, and focus on the positive aspects of the situation, your day, or your life. This is called "Selective Awareness." The traffic jam is providing you with some precious time to relax and refocus on your goals. 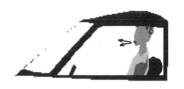 Accept the fact that you do not have any power over the traffic jam, but you do have power over how you react to it. Chill out...look for the positive!

Trains, Planes, and...!

You can try this one in the movies - or anywhere you're expected to sit for an extended period of time! Here are a few muscle power boosters for those seated events:

- Begin by checking your posture for healthy alignment. (Refer to "Sitting Rules" in the ONE-MINUTE Computer Workouts section.)

- The TRI-Umph exercises work well while seated. (Described in the ONE-MINUTE Grocery Shopping Workout section.)

- Relax your shoulders and gently lower your right ear toward your right shoulder and hold for four slow, deep breaths. Now, do the same to the left side. This stretches your neck and upper shoulder muscles (upper trapezius) and helps relieve tension in your shoulders.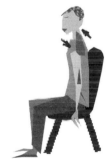

- Walk your feet in place on the floor in front of your seat. Alternate walking on your heels and then on your toes for variety.

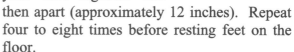

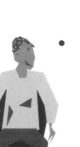

- Raise your feet slightly off the floor and bring your feet together and then apart (approximately 12 inches). Repeat four to eight times before resting feet on the floor.

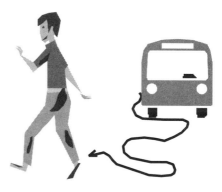

- If you commute on a bus or subway, try getting off one stop before your destination and walk the rest of the way.

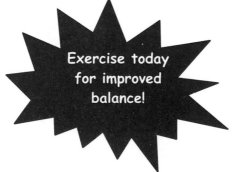

Exercise today for improved balance!

- During long train or plane commutes, practice some relaxation techniques. For example:

  - Close your eyes and clear your mind.
  - Inhale deeply, filling your diaphragm and then your lungs.
  - Exhale slowly by emptying your lungs first and then your diaphragm.
  - Continue to breathe slowly and deeply.
  - Relax your feet, calves, knees, thighs, pelvic region, abdominal muscles and lower back. Imagine all the tension flowing out of your lower body, draining out of your toes.
  - Now, relax your hands, wrists, forearms, elbows, upper arms, shoulders, chest, upper back, neck and face. Imagine all the tension flowing out of your upper body, draining out of your fingertips.
  - Allow yourself this time to relax and let the chair and floor support your entire weight.
  - After several minutes, gently rock your feet from side 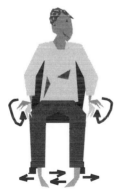 to side and slowly roll your wrists in small circles. Inhale and exhale deeply and place the palms of your hands together. Softly and then vigorously rub your palms together as you open your eyes and refocus. Remember that you are worth the time it takes to relax! We encourage you to apply this superb technique for relieving stress for your physical and psychological well being.

Planning Ahead!

When taking a trip that requires a layover, wear comfortable walking shoes and place your fashionable shoes in a carry-on bag. Now, you're set to walk away your layover and accumulate workout minutes. We also think it's more fun to "people watch" while on the move! Give it a try, we know you'll love it!

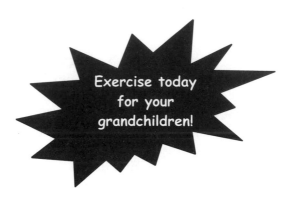

Exercise today
for your
grandchildren!

ONE-MINUTE
On-the-Job Workouts!

Fitness Fact: Holding the phone between your ear and shoulder can be the cause of chronic neck pain. If you are commonly in need of both hands while on the phone, invest in a phone adapter for your shoulder or a speaker phone.

Everyone has parts of their body in which they are satisfied and dissatisfied. Many of us tend to focus most of our attention on the body parts we don't like. Remember to celebrate the characteristics that you like and not fret about the parts of your body with which you aren't happy. Instead, focus on how you can make the most of what you are.

Select one-minute workouts in this book that highlight the areas you want to change the most. Begin with these exercises and turn your fretting into positive steps toward improving your self-esteem! This section may include several exercises that target your specific problem areas. The best part is you can do them without missing a minute of work.

There are some body parts you cannot change through exercise, for example, bone size, the size of your nose, shape of your ears. Put them in proper prospective by learning to accept them as characteristics that make you unique and special.

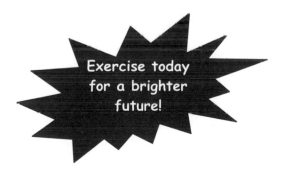
Exercise today for a brighter future!

Sorry,…. You're NOT Indispensable

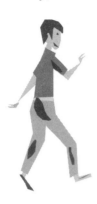

If your job requires you to sit for prolonged periods of time, get up and take a short walk in the morning, midday, and afternoon. If you must, stick to the ONE-MINUTE time frame, although we recommend turning these walks into FIVE-MINUTE workouts! Now, don't go "Type A" on us! We'll help you along. A good reason to take three short walks per day, other than your health, is to help you be more productive on the job! Really, our brains require short breaks from concentration and stress in order to function at their best. These walks will also release some mood lifting hormones, called endorphins, that will energize and prepare you for your next creative task. If you're not the type to take an aimless walk, select several walking destinations. For example, you may want to walk to your car and back, around the block, or "walk" an errand – to the post office, store, etc.

Scheduling ONE- MINUTE Workouts
If you keep a calendar or day planner at work, schedule in ONE-MINUTE workouts each day of the week. This is a fantastic way to remind yourself to get up and move throughout your workday.

Let your Feet Do the Walking
Here are some excuses to let your feet do the walking during your workday:

- Instead of using the phone, walk to your co-worker's office and discuss business matters in person. Perhaps you can even have a walking discussion.

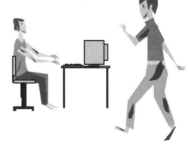

- Instead of going to the closest restroom, walk to a restroom that is located farther away. Better yet, choose a restroom on a different floor and walk some stairs.

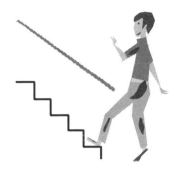

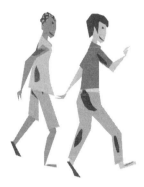

- Instead of sitting and visiting during breaks, invite a co-worker to take a walk and visit while in motion.

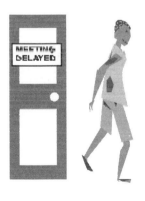

- Instead of waiting for a delayed meeting to get underway, find out how long the delay will be and take a walk to fill the time gap. No use waiting around when you can be improving your health, fitness, and mood!

Office Walking

Instead of talking on the phone while seated at your desk, get up and walk around your office! The only thing preventing you from doing this is your phone cord. Invest in an extended cord and you can add up phone fitness minutes all day long! (Walking or jogging in one place causes strain on your legs and knees. Make this a safe one-minute workout by moving <u>around</u> your office or workspace.)

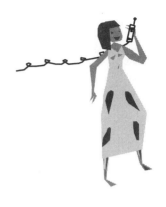

Chair Stretches

A fabulous chest (pectorals) stretch can be performed in most office chairs. While seated, simply reach your arms around the back of the chair and open your chest. This is a wonderful posture check for those who work at a desk all day!

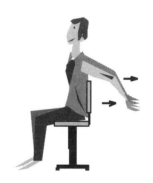

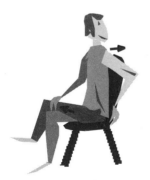

Cross your right leg over your left leg. Place your left hand on the right outer thigh and gently turn your torso to the right. Hold this position for a slow count of ten and repeat with the other leg. This stretches your outer hip (abductors) and spine region.

Sit forward in your chair and bend your right leg under the chair, balancing yourself on the ball of that foot. For support, place your hands on the bent leg. Extend your left leg straight in front of your chair. Hold this position for a slow count of ten and repeat with the other leg. This stretches the back side of your leg (hamstrings). Short, tight hamstrings can be directly related to lower back pain.

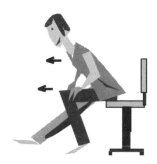

Chair Exercises

The following chair exercises are in addition to those already described in the ONE-MINUTE Out & About section (*Car Calisthenics* and *Trains, Planes, and...*):

- While seated, alternate extending your right and left legs in front of your chair. This works the front of your thighs (quadriceps).

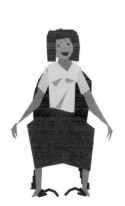

- Seated jumping jacks. Perform jumping jack feet movements (lifting feet apart and then together). This works the outer hip (abductors), inner thigh (adductors) and hip flexor muscles.

Desk Push-Ups

For a variation of the wall push-up, stand and place your hands a little more than shoulder-width apart on the edge of your desk. While supporting your weight with your extended arms, walk your feet away from the desk and perform push-ups. This works your chest (pectorals) and arms (triceps).

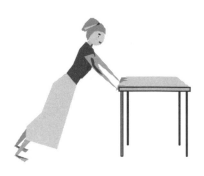

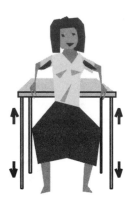

Desk Dips

No, we're not referring to a co-worker! This is another great way to work your triceps. First, make sure you are wearing non-slip shoes. Stand with your back to your desk, feet a little more than hip-width apart, with hands on the edge of the desk. Slowly lower your body into a squat position, using your arms for support, and then lift to standing position. If this is easy, extend your whole body like a ramp and perform the dips.

Co-Worker Challenges

Invite one or more of your co-workers to accept one of the following exercise challenges. Each challenge could last a week or more – it's up to you. If you're the gambling type, you might want to place a wager that involves some prize (healthy snack, lunch, etc.) for those who perform the exercises outlined in the challenge 100% of the time! This can be a hoot!

Stairs X (times) 2 - Every time you encounter a flight of stairs, walk up them, walk back down, and up again - thus, taking the stairs twice! When walking up multiple flights, we recommend you walk up, down, and back up each flight separately, rather than each direction all at once. You may want to invent your own rules for situations where many flights of stairs are involved! This exercise only takes moments out of your day, yet doubles your muscle power for this common activity.

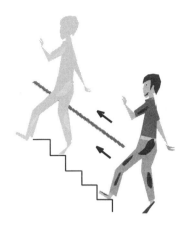

Chairs X (times) 2 – Every time you sit down in a chair, stand back up, and sit down again. This doubles your muscle power for this activity. You may have to keep an eye on your challengers! Plus, as you know, the slower you sit and stand, the better the workout!

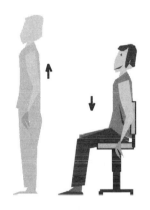

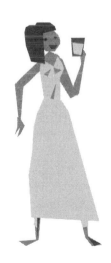

Water Watch – Everyone should have a 16 to 32 oz. plastic water bottle at work. Challenge your co-workers to drink a minimum of 32 oz. of water per day while at work. That's a mere four cups! Encourage and support one another to drink water throughout the day. Whoever doesn't buy into this healthy challenge is all wet!

ONE-MINUTE
TV Workouts!

Fitness Fact: The average American watches an equivalent of 52 days of TV a year. Every year, the average teen spends 900 hours in school and 1,500 hours watching TV. Every week, the average child between the ages of two and eleven watches 1,197 minutes of TV (that's almost 20 hours per week!). It's obvious, Americans should decrease their TV time and increase their exercise time. Turn your TV viewing into another opportunity to exercise by doing the following One-Minute TV Workouts! If you have children, turn TV watching into a family exercise event.

In this section we've provided you with a variety of "TV Workouts" from which to choose. The best part is, you can do these workouts without missing one minute of your show! All the exercises are done during the commercials. These workouts will require you to keep this book close by and refer to it at the start of each commercial break. Select a different workout each time you watch television in order to balance your program. In some cases, we've provided you with exercise intensity options. Choose the exercise with which you are most comfortable and you're ready to go!

ONE-MINUTE TV Workouts for Sculpting & Stretching Upper Body Muscles:

Before Turning on the TV: Get a glass of water and take a drink. That's a minimum of one full cup of water per drink. Turn on the set and relax.

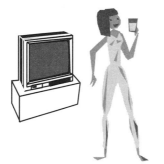

1st Commercial Break:

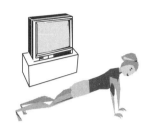

Perform eight push-ups of your choice. Choose from the following push-up difficulty levels: Most difficult = full push-ups, Moderate difficulty = modified push-ups (from the knees), Least difficult = wall push-ups. Push-ups help to strengthen your chest (pectorals) and arm (triceps) muscles. Exhale as you perform each push-up and inhale when you lower your body s-l-o-w-l-y to the start position.

2nd Commercial Break:

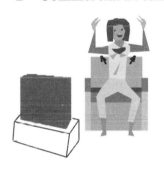

Stretch your chest (pectorals) muscles and hold for a slow count of 20. Breathe deeply as you stretch.

3rd Commercial Break:

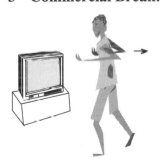

Perform four to eight shoulder blade squeezes. If you are able, perform up to three sets of eight repetitions. (Eight squeezes, short rest period, eight squeezes, short rest period, eight squeezes). This exercise is great for the upper back muscles (trapezius). Continue to breathe throughout this exercise.

4th Commercial Break:

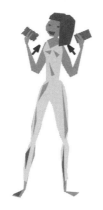

Take another drink of water (one-cup minimum), get up, re-fill your glass, and nab two food cans from the kitchen pantry or cupboard for the next commercial break.

5th Commercial Break:

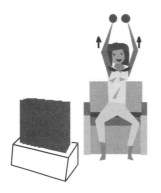

Perform four to eight kitchen can military presses. (Refer to Laundry Detergent Presses, if needed.) If you are able, perform up to three sets of eight repetitions. This exercise works the shoulders (deltoids). Exhale as you lift and inhale as you s-l-o-w-l-y lower your arms to start position.

6th Commercial Break:

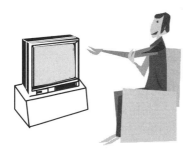

Stretch your deltoid muscles and hold each side for a slow count of 20. Breathe deeply as you stretch.

7th Commercial Break:

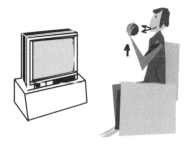

Perform four to eight kitchen can biceps curls. If you are able, perform up to three sets of eight repetitions. Exhale as you contract your biceps and inhale as you slowly relax your arms back to start position.

8th Commercial Break:

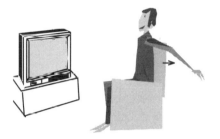

Stretch your biceps muscles and hold for a slow count of 20. Breathe deeply as you stretch.

9th Commercial Break:

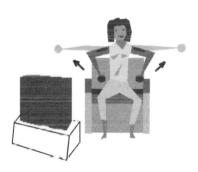

Perform four to eight kitchen can triceps extensions. If you are able, perform up to three sets of eight repetitions. Exhale as you extend your arms and inhale as you relax arms to start position.

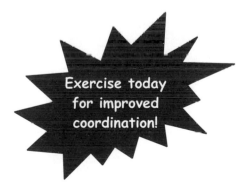

Exercise today for improved coordination!

10th Commercial Break:

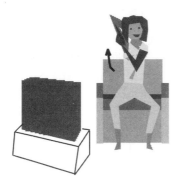

Stretch your triceps muscles and hold each side for a slow count of 20. Breathe deeply as you stretch.

Take another drink of water (one-cup minimum), get up, re-fill your glass, grab a vegetable or piece of fruit, and enjoy the rest of the show!

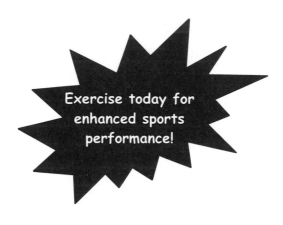

Exercise today for enhanced sports performance!

ONE-MINUTE TV Workouts for Sculpting & Stretching Lower Body Muscles:

Fitness Fact: The reason fruit juice or soda is not as good for hydration during workouts is because they are too concentrated with calories and take a longer time to empty from your stomach. Water leaves your stomach rapidly and is a much better choice for replenishing fluids quickly during and after exercise.

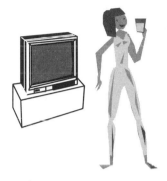

Before Turning on the TV: Get a glass of water and take a drink. That's a minimum of one full cup of water per drink. Turn on the set and relax.

1st Commercial Break:

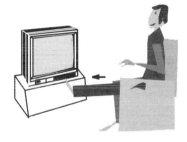

Sit tall and straighten your right and then left leg in front of your chair eight times. If you are able, repeat two more sets for a total of three sets of eight slow leg extensions. Continue to breathe during these exercises. This is an excellent exercise for the front side of your thighs (quadriceps).

2nd Commercial Break:

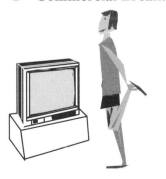

Stand or lie on your side and stretch your quadriceps muscles. Stretch each leg for a slow count of 20. Breathe deeply and never bounce into a stretch.

3rd Commercial Break:

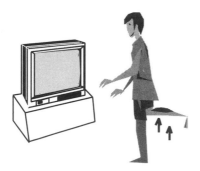

Stand and perform alternating leg curls to work the back side of your legs (hamstrings). Continue to breathe while performing a minimum of eight repetitions, or better yet, perform leg curls during the entire commercial break. WOW!

4th Commercial Break:

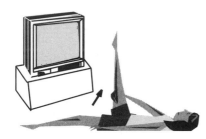

Stand, sit, or lie down and stretch your hamstrings. Stretch each leg for a slow count of 20. Breathe deeply and never bounce into a stretch.

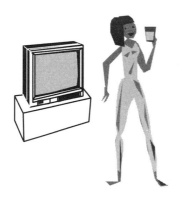

5th Commercial Break: Take another drink of water (one-cup minimum), get up and re-fill your glass.

6th Commercial Break:

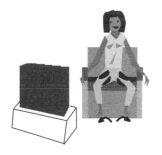

Sit tall and perform slow motion seated jumping jacks, using your legs only. This works your outer thighs (abductors, inner thighs (adductors), and hip flexor muscles. Continue to breathe and perform a minimum of eight repetitions or keep exercising throughout the entire commercial break.

7th Commercial Break:

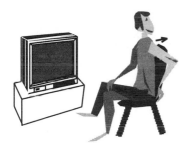

Scoot to the edge of your chair, walk your feet apart and hold this inner thigh (adductors) stretch for a slow count of twenty. Now, cross your right leg over your left leg. Place your left hand on the right outer thigh and gently turn your torso to the right. Hold this position for a slow count of ten and repeat with the other leg. This stretches your outer thigh (abductors) and spine region. Breathe deeply and never bounce into a stretch.

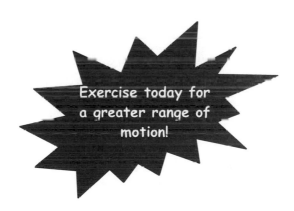

Exercise today for a greater range of motion!

8th Commercial Break:

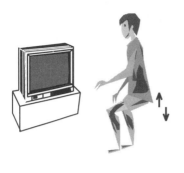

Stand and perform eight slow and controlled squats, using your hips to lower yourself as if preparing to sit down in a chair. Use good form by pushing your gluteals (buttocks) back so your knees stay behind your toes. This ensures good support for your precious knees. If you are able, perform two more sets of eight for a total of three sets of eight. Continue to breathe throughout these exercises. This works your quadriceps, hamstrings, and buttocks (gluteus maximus).

9th Commercial Break:

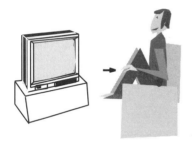

Sit or lie down and pull one or both knees toward your chest and hold for a slow count of twenty. If only stretching one leg at a time, don't forget to stretch the other side! Breathe deeply and never bounce into a stretch. This is a fabulous stretch for your gluteus maximus and lower back.

10th Commercial Break:

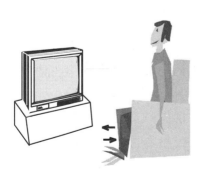

Sit tall in your chair or stand and alternate walking on your heels and toes in front of your chair. This works your calves (gastrocnemius) and shin muscles (tibialis anterior). Continue to breathe throughout these exercises.

Take another drink of water (one-cup minimum), get up, re-fill your glass, grab a vegetable or piece of fruit, and enjoy the rest of the show!

ONE-MINUTE TV Workouts for Healthy Abs & Back:

Fitness Fact: About 80% of Americans experience low back pain at some time in their lives. Giving equal time to exercises that strengthen your lower back and abdominals can often prevent this pain.

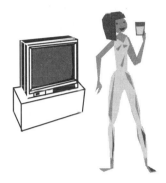

Before Turning on the TV: Go get a glass of water and take a drink. That's a minimum of one full cup of water per drink. Turn on the set and relax.

1ˢᵗ Commercial Break:

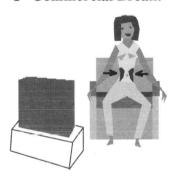

Sit tall and contract your abdominal muscles by pressing your navel (belly button) toward your spine. Breathe while holding this contraction for a slow count of four and then relax your abdominals for a count of four. Repeat for a total of eight repetitions.

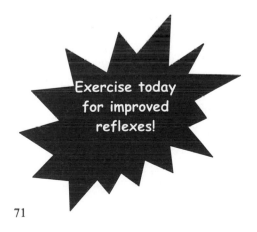

Exercise today for improved reflexes!

2nd Commercial Break:

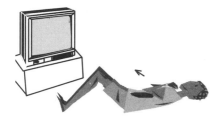

Lie down, bend your knees, and place your feet on the floor. Place your hands by your sides (easiest), across your chest (a bit harder), or lightly behind your ears with fingers open, not clasped (hardest), and slowly raise your shoulderblades off the floor. Exhale as you lift for a slow count of four and inhale as you slowly lower for another slow count of four. Repeat eight times or throughout the entire commercial break. This is working your rectus abdominus.

3rd Commercial Break:

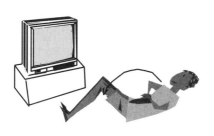

Lie on the floor in the same position as during the 2nd commercial break. This time, as you lift your shoulderblades off the floor, bring your right shoulder toward your left knee. Repeat eight times, exhaling as you lift for a slow count of four and inhaling as you lower for another slow count of four. Now, perform another eight repetitions, bringing your left shoulder toward your right knee. This works your rectus abdominus AND obliques!

4th Commercial Break:

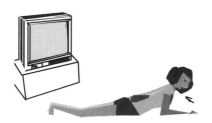

Lie on your stomach, place your elbows under your shoulders, with your forearms on the floor. Relax your head and shoulders as you slowly raise your upper body off the floor while keeping your forearms on the floor. Your hips should remain in contact with the floor at all times!

Keep breathing and hold your upper body off the floor for a slow count of eight before lowering. Repeat four times. This is an awesome stretch for your abdominal muscles while strengthening your lower back!

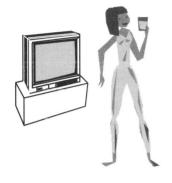

5th Commercial Break: Go take another drink of water (one-cup minimum), get up and re-fill your glass.

6th Commercial Break:

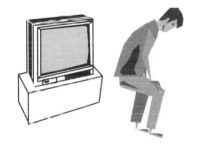

Stand with slightly bent knees (using your hips to bend), place your hands on your thighs, bring your chin toward your chest and round your back for an excellent lower back stretch. Breathe throughout this stretch.

7th Commercial Break:

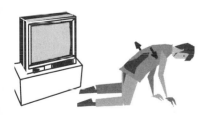

Move to the floor and place yourself on hands and knees. Bring your chin toward your chest and round your back and then lower to a flat back position. Hold each stretch for a slow count of ten and repeat four times. Continue to breathe while stretching your lower back.

8th Commercial Break:

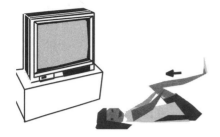

Lie on your back and bring both knees toward your chest. Hold your thighs (under your knees) and breathe through this fabulous lower back stretch. Relax your head and shoulders on the floor. Hold for a slow count of 20.

Take another drink of water (one-cup minimum), get up, re-fill your glass, grab a vegetable or piece of fruit, and enjoy the rest of the show!

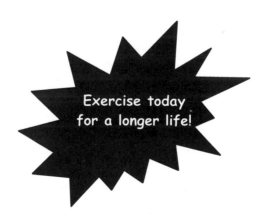

Exercise today
for a longer life!

ONE-MINUTE TV Workouts for a Healthy Heart:

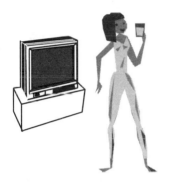

Before Turning on the TV: Get a glass of water and take a drink. That's a minimum of one full cup of water per drink. Turn on the set and relax.

1st Commercial Break:

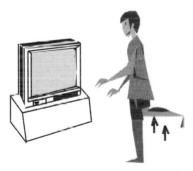

Stand and perform alternating leg curls by lifting your heel up toward your buttocks. This can be done while standing in one place or while moving around your living room or home. If you really want to pump up the action, add arm movements! Examples of arm movements include: biceps curls, pushing both arms up/out/forward and down, performing circular movements with one or both arms, swinging your arms, etc. (Turning on your own upbeat music during commercial breaks is optional!) Take a drink of water during or after every commercial break.

2nd Commercial Break:

Stand and briskly walk while mixing up the following walking patterns:

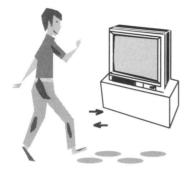

- Walk forward four steps and back four steps. Repeat four times.
- Walk with your feet apart and together, i.e., step your feet apart-apart, together-together, etc. Repeat four times.
- Walk forward two steps and back two steps. Repeat four times.
- Mix up the above walking patterns and repeat them until your minute or commercial break is over! Again, add your own arm movements if you wish to increase intensity. Water break!

3rd Commercial Break:

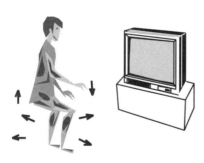

Stand, twist, and shout! You remember the twist? That's right, place one foot slightly in front of the other and swivel your hips. As you twist, lower your upright body and then raise it to add intensity. Switch your forward foot from time to time to balance the workout. Don't forget to take a drink of water.

4th Commercial Break:

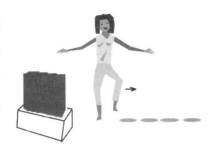

Stand and slide to the right for a count of four or eight (if you have a large room) and then to the left for a count of four or eight. Sliding is a sideways movement where you step one foot out and then slide the other foot toward it and repeat. Place your hands out to the sides for balance and be sure to lift your feet completely off the floor if sliding on carpet. We don't want you to hit a snag and take an unexpected trip. H_2O! (Water)

5th Commercial Break:

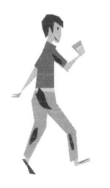

Take another drink of water (one cup minimum), get up and briskly walk to the kitchen and re-fill your glass. If time permits, extend your exercise time by briskly walking around the room or throughout your house before sitting back down.

6th Commercial Break:

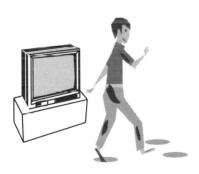

Stand and briskly walk while mixing up the following walking patterns:

- Walk forward two steps while stepping with your feet apart and then walk back two steps bringing your feet together. Your steps should form a V-pattern. Repeat four times.

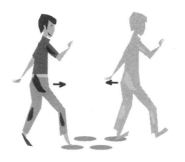

- Walk backward two steps while stepping your feet apart and then walk forward two steps bringing your feet together. Your steps should now form an inverted V-pattern. Repeat four times.

- Walk forward four steps on your toes and back four steps on your heels. Repeat four times.

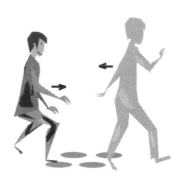

- Walk forward four steps with bent knees, lowering body; and then walk back four steps raising your body to full upright position. Repeat four times.

- Mix up the above walking patterns and repeat them until your minute or commercial break is over!

Don't forget to add your own arm movements if you wish to increase intensity. Drink, drink! (Water)

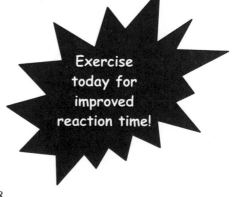

Exercise today for improved reaction time!

7th Commercial Break:

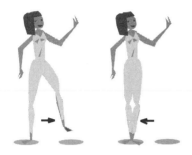

Stand and perform modified jacks by stepping your right foot out to the right and transferring your weight to the right foot. Now, bring your right foot to the start position and step your left foot to the left and transfer your weight to the left foot. Continue to step out to the right and left for a full minute or until your commercial break is over. Water break!

8th Commercial Break:

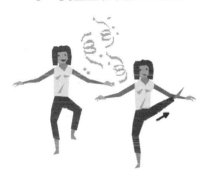

Stand and perform "Can-Cans." Lift your bent knee up and down, and then kick with the same leg. Perform this knee-lift and kick with the right leg and then the left leg. Continue repeating "can-cans" for a full minute or until your commercial break is over! Viva Las Vegas! Fill that glass of water!

9th Commercial Break:

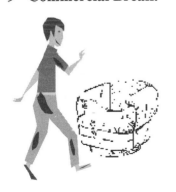

Stand and briskly walk or jog around furniture, around your room, or throughout your house during the entire commercial break. If you live in a house with stairs, don't forget to add them to your walking/jogging journey! Make sure you take a detour to the sink for a drink of water!

If you would like your *Healthy Heart TV Workouts* to continue, start at the beginning and repeat the exercises listed above. You can also add your own ideas! What about dancing to the commercial tunes, following the leader with family members, jumping an imaginary rope, skipping, walking backward, side stepping, cross-country skiing in place, etc.?

Take another drink of water (one-cup minimum), get up, re-fill your glass, grab a vegetable or piece of fruit, and enjoy the rest of the show!

Fitness Fact: The term "aerobic" was originated in the late 1960's by the Dallas, Texas, fitness expert, Dr. Kenneth Cooper.

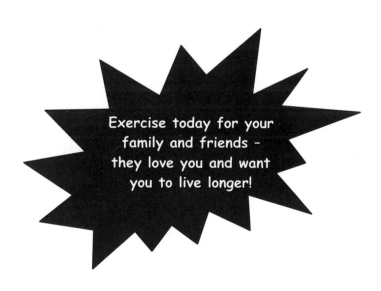

Exercise today for your family and friends – they love you and want you to live longer!

Closing Remarks

Congratulations, you are on your way to a healthier, more energetic you! We hope the exercises you have learned in this book have added "life" to your life. Now that One-Minute Workouts have become a part of your day, you'll no doubt create more lifestyle exercises of your own. Exercise should be a vital part of your life.

Being more active is an achievable goal. Keep going, prioritize exercise as a part of your daily lifestyle, and don't be surprised if people begin to say or ask you questions like...

> "You look terrific! Have you lost weight?"
> "You have so much more energy! What's your secret?"
> "You seem less stressed lately. What has changed in your life?"

Now you know that exercise, even in one-minute intervals, can help you look and feel so much better. Refer to this book from time to time and continue to add a few new exercises to your day. Remember, inch by inch, it IS a cinch! Good luck with this and all of your goals in life. Take care, stay active, and be well!

It does not matter how slowly you go,
so long as you do not stop.
- Confucius

Glossary of Key Terms

Abductors: Muscles found on your outer thighs.

Adductors: Muscles found on your inner thighs.

Aerobic Exercise: Exercise that involves large muscles of the body, is continuous, rhythmical, and requires you to breathe harder than normal – but not too hard.

Biceps: Muscles found on the front side of your upper arms.

Body Composition: The amounts of fat and lean body tissue (muscle, organs, bone) found in your body.

Cardiorespiratory Endurance: The ability of your heart and lungs to take in, transport, and utilize oxygen.

Deltoids: Muscles found in your shoulder region. Anterior Deltoids are located on the front side of your shoulders, Middle Deltoids on your upper shoulders, and Posterior Deltoids on the back side of your shoulders.

Endorphins: Hormones released during exercise that can improve your mood.

Erector Spinae: Muscles found in your lower back region.

Flexibility: The ability to move your joints through their full range of motion.

Gastrocnemius: Muscles found on your calves.

Gluteus Maximus: Muscles found on your buttocks.

Hamstrings: Muscles found on the back side of your upper legs.

Health-Related Fitness: Total health-related fitness includes the following five components – 1) cardiorespiratory endurance, 2) muscular strength, 3) muscular endurance, 4) flexibility, and 5) body composition.

Latissimus Dorsi (Lats): Large muscles found on your upper to mid-back region.

Lifestyle Activity Intervention: Incorporating exercise into your daily routine.

Metabolic Rate: The rate at which your body burns calories for energy.

Muscular Endurance: The ability of your muscles to exert force over and over again.

Muscular Strength: The maximal ability of your muscles to exert force.

Obliques: Muscles found on the outer portion of your abdominal region.

Pectoralis Major: Muscles found on your chest.

Physical Fitness: The ability to have the vitality and energy to function at an optimal level and have improved health.

Quadriceps: Muscles found on the front side of your upper legs.

Rectus Adbominis: Muscles found on your stomach.

Stress Management: The ability to effectively utilize healthy strategies to counter the negative physical effects of stress. Could be considered a sixth component of health-related fitness.

Tibialis Anterior: Muscles found on the front side of your lower legs (shins).

Trapezius: Muscles found on your upper back.

Triceps: Muscles found on the back side of your upper arms.

Index

Meet the Authors

Bonnie Nygard is a physical educator and coordinator of Physical Education & Recreation at the University of Alaska Anchorage. She has a Bachelor's degree in Physical Education and a Master's degree in Adult Education with an emphasis in Exercise Science. Bonnie developed and taught the first Fitness Leadership Certification Program in Alaska and is often seen teaching fitness classes on the Alaska Educational Television Network. In 1991, she produced and appeared in a series of award winning fitness videos. Bonnie was nominated to the Northwest AHPERD District as Alaska's University Physical Education Professional of the Year. In 1998, the University of Alaska awarded her their prestigious Chancellor's Award for Excellence in Service. Also in 1998, Bonnie Nygard and Bonnie Hopper completed the 2nd Edition of the *Innovative Fitness Connections* physical education fitness curriculum and resource package, promoting lifelong fitness habits in our youth across the country. Currently co-authoring an elementary school fitness guide, Bonnie Nygard resides in Alaska and is a highly regarded, dynamic presenter and consultant at conferences and school districts across the country.

Bonnie Hopper has a Bachelor's degree in Physical Education and a Master's degree in Education. In 1992 she was named National Elementary Physical Education Teacher of the Year. In that same year, she was profiled by Disney Channel as part of the American Teacher Awards and was the Alaska state winner and a finalist for the PTA based Phoebe A. Hearst National Educator of the Year Award. In 1998, Bonnie Hopper and Bonnie Nygard co-authored a creative and exciting physical education fitness curriculum and resource packaged called *Innovative Fitness Connections*, which is currently being used in middle and high schools across the country. Currently co-authoring an elementary school fitness guide, Bonnie Hopper resides in Montana and is a physical education consultant and motivational and enthusiastic presenter at conferences across the country.

NOV 5 2000

Books Available From Robert D. Reed Publishers

Please include payment with orders. Send indicated book/s to:

Name:_____

Address:_____

City:_____ State:_____ Zip:_____

Phone:(____)_____Fax:_____ E-mail:_____

Book Title	Unit Price	Qty.	Sub-total
Brush Strokes: A Personal Journey to Peace of Mind by Karina Berrner	$11.95	____	_____
House Calls: How we can all heal the world one visit at a time by Patch Adams, M.D.	11.95	____	_____
500 Tips For Coping With Chronic Illness by Pamela D. Jacobs, M.A.	11.95	____	_____
Coping With Your Child's Chronic Illness by Alesia T. Barrett Singer, Ph.D.	9.95	____	_____
Gotta Minute? The Ultimate Guide of One-Minute Workouts for Anyone, Anywhere, Anytime! by Nygard, M.Ed. and Hopper, M.Ed.	9.95	____	_____
Healing Is Remembering Who You Are by Marilyn Gordon, Certified Hypnotherapist	11.95	____	_____
Super Kids In 30 Minutes A Day by Karen U. Kwiatkowski, M.S., M.A.	9.95	____	_____
Get Out Of Your Thinking Box by Lindsay Collier	7.95	____	_____
Live To Be 100+ by Richard G. Deeb	11.95	____	_____
A Kid's Herb Book for Children of All Ages by Leslie Tierra, Licensed Acupuncturist	19.95	____	_____
Saving The Soul of Medicine by Margaret A. Mahony, M.D.	21.95	____	_____

Enclose a copy of this order form and payment for books. Send to address below. Shipping & handling: $2.50 for first book and $1.00 for each additional book. California residents please add 8.5% sales tax. Discounts for large orders. Please make checks payable to the publisher: Robert D. Reed. Total enclosed: $_____.

Send book orders to the publisher and contact for more information:
Robert D. Reed Publishers
750 La Playa Street, Suite 647 • San Francisco, CA 94121
Phone: (650) 994-6570 • Fax: (650) 994-6579
Email: 4bobreed@msn.com • Website: www.rdrpublishers.com